Table of Contents

Common Unhealthy Reactions of the Immune System to Substances

Types of Allergies: 7 Common Triggers, Symptoms, and More

1. Introduction to Allergies

To start things off, the 7 common allergens included in this essay's discussions will be listed below. Any other allergens not discussed here should be brought to a healthcare provider.

To better understand allergies, the following topics will be addressed in this essay: Introduction Common types of allergies Symptoms of allergies What causes allergies Factors affecting allergies Management of the condition What to do during an allergic reaction Conclusion

To define, allergies are "an overreaction of the immune system to substances that generally cause no reaction in most individuals." These substances could be anything - food, dust, pollen, pet dander, or anything else. A person who is allergic to certain substances, allergens, will have an allergic reaction once affected. This allergy's allergic reaction can be quite severe, requiring immediate medical attention.

Allergies are becoming a widespread disease, and why wouldn't they? Billions of potential allergens are present all around us, from food to pet dander, and more. In this article, we're going to look at the 7 common triggers of allergies, symptoms, and more very thoroughly.

2. Understanding the Immune System and Allergic Reactions

Under most circumstances, this is an admirable trait. It ensures that you remain safe. However, your immune system's hypersensitivity can be one of these traits that play a role. For instance, at the whiff of a harmless substance, such as pet dander (tiny flakes of skin that cats, dogs, and other animals shed), your immune system may go a little overboard and turn the professional allergy alarm on. And that sets off a chain of events in your body. This is what's happening in your system if you're sneezing, coughing, or wheezing because you have allergies. Note: What exactly is occurring in the body can be difficult to understand. This is why this article is intended to provide you with some foundational information to help improve your understanding of allergies and sensitivities, immune reactions, and other topics.

Your body's intricate system designed to fight off invaders and infections is called your immune system. It prevents illness and infection by seeking and destroying dangerous pathogens such as bacteria, viruses, parasites, and fungi. To summarize, this network of cells, tissues, and organs is designed to work together to keep you healthy. Your immune system can identify and remember specific pathogens and rapidly eliminate them the next time it detects them in your body. The cells of the immune system are appropriately designed to fight off harmful substances, such as infections.

3. Types of Allergies

- Respiratory allergies: These are sometimes called environmental allergies. Common triggers are airborne substances, such as pollen, animal dander, and mold; they can be exacerbated and act as actual allergens. - Food allergies: These occur when the body has a specific type of immunologic response to a specific ingredient; most reactions result because of proteins. - Eosinophilic conditions: These include symptoms similar to those associated with allergies, but the reaction involves proinflammatory cells. - Skin allergies: These can cause allergies when the skin comes into contact with a specific food or substance, as this is a nonsystemic reaction. - Medication allergies: These arise as a result of an immunologic reaction due to a prescribed medication or one you can buy without a prescription. Any medicine can cause an allergy, but some medications more commonly cause allergic reactions. - Insect stings: Bee or wasp stings more commonly cause allergic reactions, which result from the venom injected into your body by the insect. - Latex allergy: Rubber products, such as medical and surgical gloves, have led to asthma, hand dermatitis, and hives with some people; your risk of exposure to rubber increases if you work in the health care field.

There are several types of allergies. Some stem from contact with allergens like pollen or molds, while others are triggered by irritants that also cause symptoms similar to certain allergies. Allergies can be mild, such as causing a rash or hives, or severe, such as leading to anaphylaxis. No matter what type of allergy you have, medications or treatments reduce allergy symptoms.

The main triggers for respiratory allergies are dust mites, mold, cockroaches, tree pollen, grass pollen, and ragweed pollen, as well as animal dander and mold spores that may trigger allergic asthma. Medical treatment for respiratory allergies includes over-the-counter and prescription medications like antihistamines, decongestants, and corticosteroids. Additionally, people with respiratory allergies may be able to get relief by using saline rinses, performing other forms of nasal irrigation, and using an over-the-counter wash like Allergon before bed. The general term for respiratory allergies is allergic rhinitis, which literally translates to irritated nose. It is characterized by sneezing, itching, a runny nose, nasal congestion, a sensation of a wet rue, and stuffy or full feeling in the nose.

An allergic reaction of the respiratory system, respiratory allergies can range from relatively mild to serious and chronic. Though symptoms of a respiratory allergy can come out of the blue, people tend to suffer more of these allergic reactions during certain times of the year. For instance, plants, grass, and trees are all known to produce pollen, which can lead to more allergic reactions in North America during the spring. Additionally, many respiratory allergies are referred to as atopic disorders and can run in families; data suggest when one parent has an atopic disorder like a respiratory allergy, children have a 1-in-2 to 2-in-3 chance of acquiring one, either. On the whole, most respiratory allergies and atopic disorders can be effectively managed.

3.2. 2. Food Allergies

A certified allergist can diagnose a food allergy, beginning with a physical examination and detailed patient history. Treatment recommendations may include: oral corticosteroids for GI swelling; antihistamines to reduce hives and oral itching, rashes, and GI symptoms; and epinephrine for anaphylaxis. Appropriate nutrition is crucial because a safe and well-balanced diet can prevent GI symptoms. In severe cases, elimination diets, in which common allergens are removed for a period of time and then added back into the diet one at a time, can help patients to become their best advocate. Extreme caution should be exercised when handling food and cooking in order to prevent a major allergic outbreak.

Managing Food Allergy Symptoms

In a patient with IBS, a food allergen can trigger symptoms associated with the disease. Those with known allergy issues should talk to their gastroenterologists to see if the allergen has any connection with their IBS.

Secondary Irritable Bowel Syndrome (IBS)

Symptom severity can vary case-by-case, but food allergies can manifest as a collection of symptoms that affect the skin, gastrointestinal (GI) system, and even the respiratory system. It's also possible to experience dizziness and a rapid or weak pulse as well as anaphylactic symptoms. The skin may get red and swollen, ending in a breakout of hives, considered a classic allergy symptom. Additionally, an allergen can cause irritation of the esophagus (the tube that connects the throat and stomach, and has a muscular action to move food to the stomach), and other areas within the GI system.

Food Allergy Symptoms

- Milk - Peanuts - Tree nuts, such as walnuts - Fish - Shellfish - Eggs - Soy - Wheat

The most common food allergens that trigger immune responses conducive to an allergic reaction include:

Food Allergy Triggers

Food Allergies

3.3. 3. Skin Allergies

Diagnosis To find out exactly what is causing the allergic reaction will be a test. Allergy testing might involve skin testing. This means a small amount of a possible allergen is placed under the surface of the skin or on the surface of the skin, which is then pricked to allow the substance to get under the skin. If a person is allergic, a reaction which leads to swelling, redness, and itching might occur. It's your body's natural response to get rid of or protect against a foreign product. Blood tests such as RAST (radioallergosorbent test) might be ordered to test for antibodies or a chemical that is released in larger reactions.

Symptoms Common signs and symptoms of skin allergies include: rash, redness, itching, hives. These symptoms can be mild but will usually be very severe and have a big impact on a person's life.

What causes skin allergies? - Dry skin, which can lead to eczemas - Dyes used in makeup, fabrics, and other materials - Hair dyes - The glue used in sticking artificial nails - Latex used to make rubber gloves, balloons, and other materials - Metals like nickel, which is found in coins and costume jewelry - Perfumes found in soaps, shampoos, and other products - The sun, giving us a rash in places that have been exposed to sunlight - Poison ivy, oak, or sumac

What are skin allergies? Skin allergies are of various kinds: some can be brief, others can be chronic, affecting the quality of life.

3.4. 4. Insect Sting Allergies

Prevention: It is done through complete eradication of potential insect stingers from the home setting, venom immunotherapy, and self-administered epinephrine devices. Identification and avoidance of potential insect stingers, picnic area hazards, and knowledge of individual diagnosis are essential in minimizing the risk associated with hymenoptera stings. After an allergic reaction, a doctor may do allergy testing, and venom immunotherapy or allergy shots are available to reduce your risk of future attacks.

Management: An insect sting allergy is an emergency. Seek immediate medical help. Desensitization through venom immunotherapy is often necessary for successful treatment of insect sting allergies. Medications are also used to reduce inflammation and for symptomatic relief.

Symptoms: Mild local reaction at sting site, chronic hives, mild to severe angioedema, severe systemic symptoms of urticaria, dizziness, wheezing, nausea, vomiting, diarrhea, abdominal pain, stridor, incapacitation, and hypotension are seen most commonly with yellow jacket hypersensitivity. Anaphylactic reactions entail upper- and lower-respiratory compromise, pruritic, urticarial, lighted redness, and warmth of the skin are more common in adults than children.

Insect stings are quite common and usually cause minor discomfort and redness around the sting region. However, in some cases, a person may have a severe allergic reaction to the venom injected by the insect. The most common stinging insects found around the house are hornets, yellow jackets, wasps, and bees belonging to the genus Apis. A person with insect sting allergy may have a generalized reaction to the sting. The reactions range from mild lip swelling to severe wheezing and hypotension. The allergic reactions are often because of the substances: melitin, hyaluronidase, histamine, phospholipase, and proteases present in insect venom.

Section 3: Type of Allergy 3.4.4. Insect Sting Allergies

3.5. 5. Drug Allergies

5. Drug Allergies An allergy to a particular drug or medication is called a drug allergy. A hyperactive response to a drug is what causes a drug allergy. They might not have a reaction while consuming the drug, but if they consume it later, they may. The symptoms of medication allergies may occur on the skin, such as itching and skin rashes. Other signs and symptoms include swelling of the face, eyes, or lips, wheezing, coughing, or shortness of breath, fainting or weakness, and so on. In adults, nonsteroidal anti-inflammatory drugs (NSAIDs) such as ibuprofen or aspirin, two groups of antibiotics, sulfa drugs, and penicillin, are the most prevalent causes of drug allergies. Drug allergies can usually be confirmed through skin testing or detection of IgE antibodies. Oral drug challenges and other drug-specific testing might be required for a negative skin result.

You can also include other information such as different courses of therapy and management for drug allergies. Elucidating the resemblances and the differences could provide a comprehensive understanding of the similarity in dealing with other kinds of allergies and the specificity of handling drug allergies. Finally, presenting the review on preventive measures, the role of physicians, and some exemplification from previous patients may complete the topic in a more engaging way.

This section of the topic discusses the other kinds of allergies, distinguishing it as the allergies triggered by certain drugs or medications. Contrary to the negative effects of taking these drugs in the form of allergic symptoms, delivering types of cure or relief could also be the main concern for the medical plan. Providing information about the symptoms of drug allergies, going deeper with the medical diagnosis to ensure the causality of the drugs themselves would be very useful for the audience that seek such health information.

4. Common Triggers of Allergies

There are also allergic and non-allergic forms of a disease called eosinophilic esophagitis that is of interest to the members of our group. People with eosinophilic esophagitis can have problems with swelling and constriction in their esophagus. It can be caused by chronic allergic inflammation from food, which is called allergic eosinophilic esophagitis, or it can be from some other cause, which is non-allergic eosinophilic esophagitis. A person can also have other symptoms such as food allergies, environmental allergies, or allergic reactions in their skin or blood. These people may have what is now called a type 2 inflammatory disease. In these diseases, there are special types of cells called eosinophils and mast cells that are in the body in high numbers, and they are making some chemicals called cytokines, chemotactic factors, and lipid-like molecules that can cause harm to the body.

About a third of people with asthma have eosinophilic asthma. Eosinophils are a type of white blood cell. There are a few different kinds of diseases and conditions that can cause people to have too many eosinophils in their body. These conditions are called eosinophilic disorders. One of these eosinophilic disorders is eosinophilic granulomatosis with polyangiitis. It used to be known as Churg-Strauss syndrome. People with this disease have a history of asthma, sinusitis, nose polyps, and allergic reactions on their skin.

Insect stings Many different types of bug bites can cause allergic reactions, but a sting from a honeybee, yellow jacket, wasp, hornet, or fire ant can cause serious life-threatening problems. Medications such as penicillin and other antibiotics, aspirin and nonsteroidal anti-inflammatory drugs such as ibuprofen, can also cause allergies. An allergist/immunologist can help identify and treat the cause of reactions.

From bread and nuts to fish and milk, foods can cause allergic reactions in some people. Nine foods cause 90% of food reactions in the United States. They are milk, egg, peanut, tree nuts, wheat, soy, fish, and shellfish.

From pollens to pet dander and seasonal changes, there are many things in our environment that can trigger plant allergies. For example, dust mites, mold, and dog and cat dander can all cause sniffles and sneezes, itchy watery eyes, difficulty breathing, wheezing, and rashes. In children and babies, triggers can also include cockroaches, which can be found in urban homes, mold, animal hair, food, dust mites, and atopic dermatitis.

4.1. 1. Environmental Triggers

While there are many allergens out there, certain ones are much more common than others. Here's an overview of the most common environmental triggers and the allergies they can stimulate. These triggers are common culprits behind hay fever, or allergic rhinitis. That common allergic condition affects about 1 in 5 people, according to the Centers for Disease Control and Prevention (CDC), and is characterized by a constellation of symptoms that typically affect the upper respiratory tract. Minimizing exposure to environmental triggers in and around your home may help you manage your symptoms.

Environmental triggers, specifically common allergens present in the environment, often provoke an allergic reaction. These could be airborne pollutants like dust, mold, and pet hair. If you're a sufferer of allergies, you might fret a new bout of sneezing, coughing, or itchy eyes every time you go outside or gather up an old book. It's generally not possible or widely feasible, however, to avoid these triggers entirely. In part, that's because they're found around the whole world and in homes and other buildings. Allergens can also pollute air and even drinking water, affecting us as we move through our daily routines. Instead, doctors usually recommend symptom management or medicines that might lessen their impacts. They might also suggest setting up a game plan to keep yourself away from these triggers as much as possible.

Managing and treating a food allergy depends on how severe the reaction is and how much of the allergen the person was exposed to. In the U.S., there is no medication that can cure a food allergy, unlike the idea of medication for an upset stomach or food poisoning. However, antihistamines can control symptoms for mild to moderate attacks. There is also a risk of a delayed allergic reaction that occurs within 24 to 72 hours called a "food intolerance," which also raises concerns.

Final Thoughts

Some of the most prevalent food allergens include milk, eggs, fish, shellfish, tree nuts, peanuts, wheat, and soybeans. More than 170 foods are reported to cause allergic reactions, according to the Food and Drug Administration (FDA). In total, inadequate digestion leads to problems in both macro- and micronutrients. Digestive enzyme imbalances have been shown to increase inflammation, and altered gut flora cause gut mucosa damage. This inappropriate handling consequently leads to the development of various gastrointestinal symptoms, including gas, bloating, nausea and/or vomiting, abdominal discomfort, diarrhea and/or constipation, and irritable bowel diseases. If continued exposure occurs, these acute symptoms contribute to another intrinsic pathology characterized by abdominal pain, difficulty swallowing and/or breathing, and hives, urticaria, and/or angioedema. This effect leads to a serious life-threatening condition known as anaphylaxis, marked by low blood pressure, respiratory or cardiac arrest, and/or seizure, resulting in fatal outcomes. Managing and treating a food allergy depends on how severe the reaction is and how much of the allergen the person was exposed to. In the U.S., there is no medication that can cure a food allergy, unlike the idea of medication for an upset stomach or food poisoning. However, antihistamines can control symptoms for mild to moderate attacks. There is also a risk of a delayed allergic reaction that occurs within 24 to 72 hours called a "food intolerance," which also raises concerns.

Common Food Triggers

4.3. 3. Insect Stings

"For those who are allergic or suspect they could be allergic to insect stings, the safest approach is to be evaluated by an allergist," Lambrecht says. "If a severe allergy is confirmed, then the provider can discuss measures, including the use of epinephrine auto-injectors and possibly venom immunotherapy, to reduce the risk of a severe allergic reaction to insect stings in the future." Preventing insect stings is the first line of defense against an insect sting allergy. Some ways to reduce the risk of being stung include: - Avoiding being barefoot in grassy areas or near garbage cans or beer cans - Wearing long sleeves and pants when doing yard work - Avoiding floral-patterned clothing, perfumes, scented lotions, and hair sprays when spending long periods of time outdoors - Keeping windows and doors closed, especially in below-grade areas, so that stinging insects cannot build nests.

Insect stings Reactions to insect stings are common, affecting 5% of the population in the United States, according to the AAAAI. Most stinging insects in the United States belong to one of three groups: bees, wasps, or ants. For individuals allergic to certain insect venoms, being stung can cause a severe allergic reaction called anaphylaxis. An allergic reaction to stings from these insects can occur at any time, even if stings from the same insect were tolerated in the past. "The vast majority of people are not allergic to these insect venoms and will have only uncomfortable but uneventful localized reactions when stung," says Dr. LaPook. "However, if you're allergic, your immune system reacts to the allergens in the sting's venom in a way that is harmful to your own body, causing anaphylaxis."

4.4. 4. Medications

The most common allergy-causing medications include sulfa drugs, penicillin, and non-steroidal anti-inflammatory medications. For any existing skin or mucous membrane rashes, antihistamines may be helpful. If the condition is more severe, a doctor will often prescribe an oral corticosteroid. If your throat starts to close or it's hard for you to breathe, use an EpiPen if one is prescribed, and contact emergency responders immediately (Dial 911). Note that antihistamines cannot effectively reverse anaphylaxis.

Allergy to these drugs has not been well documented but may occur more frequently than previously thought. Some of the symptoms of a drug allergy include hives, itching, respiratory symptoms (chest congestion, chest pain, wheezing, and shortness of breath), or cardiovascular symptoms (dizziness or faintness). It is also possible to have anaphylaxis, the most severe allergic reaction. In anaphylaxis, a patient develops swelling of the throat, with a sudden onset of breathing difficulties accompanied by a sudden drop in blood pressure.

NSAIDs. Aspirin, ibuprofen (like Advil and Motrin), and naproxen are some of the most well-known NSAIDs. They can provoke both mild and severe reactions, including hives, generalized itching, swelling of the throat, and life-threatening anaphylaxis.

Opioids. Morphine, codeine, Vicodin, and Percocet are the most common prescription opioids, and they can trigger mild to severe skin reactions or anaphylactic shock.

Penicillin and penicillin-family drugs. Symptoms of a penicillin allergy can range from a skin rash to difficulty breathing. The severity of the reaction can worsen with each subsequent dose of the antibiotic. Fortunately, a penicillin allergy test can offer insight into whether you're truly allergic. If you're not, it's best to undergo desensitization therapy, if you still need the antibiotic, rather than avoiding it. That said, not all scenarios require desensitization, which is why it's important to consult an allergist for a proper evaluation.

Make sure you know what you're allergic to, so you can keep a running list of the things you should avoid. The most common medications that cause allergic reactions include:

Medications

5. Symptoms of Allergies

A less severe but important food allergy with gastrointestinal (primarily oral) symptoms is an allergic reaction to a protein in raw fruits and vegetables, known as oral allergy syndrome (OAS). Approximately one-third of individuals with allergic rhinitis have OAS. Symptoms include itching and some other symptoms in the mouth, and there is no risk of life-threatening anaphylaxis. The signs and symptoms of allergies can appear quickly after exposure to an allergen, or they can develop over time. Allergic reactions can range in severity, from mild to severe. Gastrointestinal symptoms in food-allergic individuals might also suggest an allergic basis if present when other body systems are not involved. Such symptoms include distension and discomfort, without diarrhea or cramping. The range of allergy symptoms is from mild to severe, and they vary from person to person. In some individuals, allergies can trigger allergic asthma or make them more reactive to environmental triggers such as tobacco smoke, pollution, or cold air.

One of the most common types of allergies is an allergy related to the respiratory system. Various allergens can mimic the symptoms of the common cold or cause attacks of asthma (reversible narrowing of the airways). Common allergies related to the respiratory system include allergic rhinitis (hay fever), allergic conjunctivitis (eye irritation), sinus infection, cough, wheezing, and shortness of breath. Allergic reactions can also cause a rash (known as eczema).

The rash is red, itchy, and scaly, and it can blister and weep. Allergies with gastrointestinal symptoms make up one category of a group of food-associated disorders. The primary allergic gastrointestinal component is food protein-induced enterocolitis syndrome (FPIES).

5.1. 1. Respiratory Symptoms

3. 5.1. 1. 2.2. Adverse food reactions An adverse food response or intolerance may sometimes mimic the symptoms of an allergy but is less damaging to the body. Lactose intolerance is a classic example of an intolerance. Since the body stops producing lactase, the enzyme that helps it digest lactose sugar, these people develop a wide range of symptoms from exposure to dairy food. They might have the same symptoms as an allergy sufferer, such as a stomach upset, cramps, and diarrhea, but those symptoms are not caused by an immune response. People with intolerances might find that symptoms resolve when they reduce or remove a specific food or foods from their diets.

2. 5.1. 1. 2.1. Food Allergies A food allergy is when one's body's immune system reacts in an extreme manner to one or more proteins in a kind of food. The trigger for most severe food allergies is any of the Big 8 foods.

D. Medications - Nasal corticosteroids: Nasal corticosteroids are corticosteroids specifically for the nose. - Antihistamine nasal sprays: Antihistamine nasal sprays are nasal decongestion sprays that include antihistamines. - Decongestants: Decongestants minimize nasal congestion by shrinking blood vessels. However, this medicine should not be taken for long periods of time. It can lead to side effects such as a rebound effect, dependency, and congestion.

C. Diagnosis - Through a physical examination. - Analysis of the patient's medical history. - The doctor might ask the patient if his or her family has had allergies. - In addition, the doctor may use allergy skin testing to identify the allergen that is causing the symptoms.

B. Effects on individuals Since the nose and sinuses are the body's natural air purifiers, when individuals are exposed to triggers, these mucous-lined organs will overreact, causing the symptoms.

A. Signs - A runny nose - A cough - Sore throat - Itchy, watery red eyes - Wheezing - Shortness of breath

5.2. 2. Skin Symptoms

These kinds of skin symptoms can occur during certain times of the year, such as during the height of pollen season, if you're allergic to tree, grass, or weed pollens. If you're allergic to substances like pet dander or dust mites that are in your everyday living environment, you could develop skin symptoms at any time. It's rare, however, for people to be exposed to an allergen by touching it and develop skin symptoms. If you do, you've likely inhaled the allergen and then transferred it to your skin by touching a surface it settled on. In order to develop any type of allergy, you must first be sensitized to that substance. The immune system of someone with hay fever, for example, is overly sensitive to pollen. The first time you were exposed to that particular type of pollen, your body responded by developing immune cells that could identify the pollen if it entered your system again.

- Itchy or red skin - Hives, or raised red welts on the skin - Dermatitis, or a skin rash that can turn scaly or develop blisters - Prurigo nodules, which are bumpy sores that can resemble bug bites - Swelling in the face, lips, hands, or arms

One of the most common complaints allergy sufferers have is an itchy rash. The changes in your immune system caused by your allergies can trigger these itchy episodes, leading to a variety of different skin symptoms. These include:

5.3. 3. Gastrointestinal Symptoms

Gastrointestinal symptoms develop at different times after the ingestion of the allergen in different people. In many cases, an allergic reaction will not begin until two hours or more after ingesting the offending food. In some people, allergies are more likely to produce symptoms when food is ingested in a large quantity or on an empty stomach. In addition, transportation of food into the body from the stomach may slow down, delaying digestion of the meal. Since food digestion may be slower moving through the body, it is thought that the immune cells in the intestines have a longer "window of opportunity" to be activated. If this happens, the immune system can produce an allergic reaction to the food.

The gastrointestinal system can be affected by food allergies and environmental allergies, such as oral allergy syndrome. Gastrointestinal symptoms may include vomiting, diarrhea, stomach pain, cramping, gas, bloating, belching, and a "heavy" feeling in the stomach. These symptoms are usually easy to manage after identifying underlying food allergies and environmental allergens. Contact a doctor for testing and management if you are experiencing any of these symptoms. Notably, symptoms of a food allergy can extend beyond the gastrointestinal system. For example, a fish allergy may cause diarrhea, breathing difficulties, and hives. On the other hand, a pollen allergy may cause your mouth to itch while or after eating a food related to that pollen.

6. Diagnosis of Allergies

Allergists/immunologists are specialists who often diagnose and manage allergies. Family physicians, pediatricians, or other healthcare providers may also manage allergies, but they may not have the extensive training of an allergist/immunologist. Allergists/immunologists with experience in treating allergies and asthma are best suited to diagnose and treat your allergic disease. Your allergy treatment will be based on your symptoms and how severe they are. It may include three different treatment strategies: avoidance of allergens, medication options, and/or immunotherapy (allergy shots). An allergist/immunologist has advanced training and experience to determine what treatment is best for you and to implement such treatment. With the right treatment plan, you can reduce or eliminate sensitivity to your allergens, experience fewer symptoms and complications, and enjoy a better quality of life.

Blood test: Also called Radioallergosorbent Test (RAST). Measures the immune system's response to common allergens. Your results will reveal how severe your allergies are. Skin test: Puts a tiny amount of the allergen just under the skin with a needle. If you are allergic to the substance, you will develop redness, swelling, and itching at the test site within 20 minutes. Once your allergens have been identified, your healthcare provider can teach you ways to reduce your exposure to them and provide allergy medication.

After discussing your personal and family medical history as well as your current symptoms, a medical professional will recommend an allergy test to determine the cause of your reactions. There are four different types of allergy tests:

6.1. 1. Allergy Testing Methods

The most common types of allergy tests are skin prick tests and blood tests. Patch tests are used to diagnose delayed contact dermatitis from substances that people come into contact with daily, such as preservatives, dyes, metals, rubber, medications, and fragrances. Many allergens measured in both allergen skin prick tests (type I IgE-mediated) and allergen blood tests (type I and/or type II T-cell mediated) are measured subjectively and/or qualitatively. It is essential to use allergy tests (skin prick tests and blood tests) to identify which allergens are important and may be triggers of their allergic disease. Furthermore, the tests can be quantitatively and objectively measured. It is important to perform allergy tests in the "allergy diagnosis" to identify which allergens, if tested positive, may need to be included in avoiding parameters - allergen reduction in the environment. It is important to identify which allergens are positive in an allergy test to establish the potential impact of allergy treatment. Given this, it must be emphasized that in achieving a diagnosis of allergy, allergy tests should always be performed simultaneously with taking medical histories (clinical presentations and allergy symptoms).

An allergy test is a type of test performed by an allergist or medical provider to determine if a person has an allergic reaction to a specific substance. An allergen is a trigger for the immune system or allergy antibody (IgE) responsible for allergic reactions. Inhaled allergens are found in the environment from things such as feathers, animal dander (from skin, fur, or feathers), molds, fungi, and certain food allergens in certain sensitivity types.

6.2. 2. Consultation with an Allergist

Life-threatening issues can arise as a result of allergies. As a result, it is important to consult an allergist to confirm and control allergies. You can always consult an allergist if you suspect you have developed an allergy, no matter if you have already started medication. Just because a symptom, such as a runny nose, cropped up, doesn't mean you should ignore the seasonal allergen. "There are various ways to feel in the body whether it is an allergy to a certain substance or not. To some people, the common perception is that smelling the source causes extreme discomfort while they won't feel a thing because impaired allergic smell prevents it, based on the predilection area. There are allergic symptoms without sniffles or rashes in other ways, such as heart problems, discomfort at the level of bronchial asthma, swelling of the glands, or changes in body balance. The allergist will be able to diagnose and treat a range of allergic conditions."

Patients must consult allergists when they suspect they have allergies. It is impossible to cure but can be controlled with the help of the allergist. The allergist will conduct a skin or blood test to confirm if the allergen is causing a cold to the patient. The allergist will then make a treatment plan based on this, which includes medicines and the necessary advice.

7. Treatment Options for Allergies

Immunotherapy: Allergy shots or sublingual tablets may be an effective treatment option for your allergy if your allergies are moderate to severe (e.g. year-round rhinitis, moderate to severe allergic seasonal asthma, venom allergy, or pet allergy) and/or you have failed or are intolerant of medications that would correct or manage your condition. Immunotherapy can also help to reduce the number of new allergies that develop and the worsening of other allergies, in addition to improving allergy symptoms and reducing medication use (up to 80 percent). Immunotherapy consists of repeat injections of progressively stronger dosages of a vaccine that is composed of extracts of allergens to which the person is allergic. It can have a significant duration of efficacy, even after the injections are ended and done for at least three to five years. After testing and examination, make an appointment with the allergist for information on allergen immunotherapy.

Allergen avoidance: It is important to identify and avoid offending allergens, if possible, to minimize exposure that may lead to your allergy symptoms. This may mean making some changes in your lifestyle or work environment. For instance, asthma patients who have dust mite allergies may notice an improvement in their symptoms from using an allergy-proof mattress cover and pillow, installing a high-efficiency filter in their residence, and washing linens weekly in hot water.

Pharmacologic treatments: Treatments with medications that benefit most people who have allergies (outside of anaphylaxis) include daily corticosteroid nasal sprays, non-drowsy OTC antihistamines, leukotriene receptor antagonists, and antihistamine eye drops.

For those who have allergies, the outlook is not as bleak as it used to be. There are many effective medications that may help you control your symptoms. Additionally, a variety of other treatments may offer you relief from your allergies, including medications, allergen avoidance (in the right scenarios), and immunotherapy. These treatments all have a place in managing your allergies. The severity of your allergic disease, as well as your test results and/or the nature of your symptoms, will all be factors in determining which treatment(s) would be right for you.

7.1. 1. Medications

Being informed and working closely with an allergist can help you make a personalized plan that's right for you. Whether you or your child has seasonal, year-round, food, or another type of allergy, the following factors can help inform your treatment.

3 Factors to Consider When Deciding to Take Allergy Medications

- Antihistamines: Various over-the-counter (OTC) and prescription antihistamine options are available to treat allergy symptoms ranging from hay fever to hives and more. - Corticosteroids: Both short-term and long-term corticosteroids are used to manage allergic reactions, including skin reactions, nasal symptoms, asthma, and more. - Mast cell stabilizers: These preventative allergy medications can help reduce the frequency and severity of allergic reactions. Examples include ketotifen, lodoxamide, and cromolyn. - Leukotriene modifiers: These medications block leukotrienes, substances in the body that contribute to seasonal allergies, asthma, and other allergic conditions. - Omalizumab (Xolair): Omalizumab can help prevent allergy symptoms in people who have asthma or chronic hives where other treatments haven't been helpful.

The most common medications are:

An allergist may prescribe or recommend several types of medications for you or your child's allergies. The treatment plan typically involves medications for both short-term relief and long-term control. For example, if you're among the millions of Americans who experience spring allergies, your doctor may prescribe antihistamines to manage a runny nose, sneezing, and itchy, watery eyes. People with food allergies who have accidentally eaten something they're allergic to may also need emergency epinephrine.

Medications

1.2 A Few Concepts It's important to grasp the significance of environmental control. It's not possible to eliminate all airborne allergens from inside the home. There is no "hypoallergenic dog" or "cat." Cats may create more allergen per kilogram of weight than dogs. Rising globally, the effects of pollen can be difficult to manage, depending on individual immune reaction diversity. Because forcing living things out of their native habitat can have unanticipated effects, recapture should never be tried. While domestic animals are the principal cause for many, more productive strategies for pet separation and possession issues are available. Social issues involving diverse needs should be taken into consideration when examining environmental controls.

1.1 Environmental Control An allergist can help pinpoint the specific allergens contributing to allergic reactions and propose environmental control measures for those circumstances. Environmental control recommendations can vary from person to person. A single allergen may be a modest component of allergen avoidance for a single person, but it may be a major issue for someone else. Because allergen avoidance can be cumulative, removing a variety of allergens simultaneously can be beneficial. For certain allergens, simple house cleaning can be sufficient. For primary household dust mites, for example, the American College of Allergy, Asthma & Immunology (ACAAI) recommends washing bedding in hot water once a week and covering pillows and mattresses with dust-proof covers. Animals are one of the most common causes of indoor allergens. Some homes are designed with flooring spaces, and some people may need to install particular air filters to reduce airborne furry allergens.

Sometimes it's impossible to avoid these triggers, but in other cases, the risk of an allergic reaction can be minimized through strategies. One environmental control method involves reducing your exposure to certain allergens. This is called allergen avoidance. For many, allergen avoidance can be an effective approach to prevent or reduce the impact of allergic reactions.

3. Immunotherapy Immunotherapy (also known as 'allergy shots') has been around for nearly a century and is regarded as the only 'disease-modifying' treatment for allergies. As both academy and industry are constantly refining its methods, allergy researchers are still looking for the point at which someone can discontinue treatment and remain immunologically desensitized, also known as interruption, and at the optimal protocol for delivering this type of intervention. 'The modern approach to immunotherapy is to give an increasing dose of the patient's antigens, which is what the relevant allergens are,' Sweer said. 'Early on, you're really only getting a very, very small amount, but it gradually and incrementally increases so your immune system stops fighting it so much.' More recently, in addition to parenteral-based immunotherapy, the newer practice of sublingual immunotherapy (SLIT), in which progressive doses of the allergenic substance are placed under the tongue, has come increasingly into use, though it has been more slow to be taken up by U.S. practitioners until recently. In the case of some environmental causes such as pollen, drops can be taken daily during the allergy season.

New research involving SLIT treatments may help increase the convenience and complete uptake of this treatment and may generate increased interest in and acceptance of this approach. Immunotherapy with venom, pollen, dust mite, and other environmental allergens works by progressively administering tiny, increasing quantities of the allergen to which someone is allergic, so their body can become better adjusted to it. Many treatment options can be used to address allergies. Over-the-counter and prescription medications can help relieve symptoms, and avoiding allergens can help prevent symptoms from occurring in the first place. Immunotherapy is another treatment option that can actually desensitize someone who is allergic to an allergen, making it less likely that they will have a severe reaction to it. Immunotherapy gradually exposes someone to increasing amounts of an allergen over time, decreasing their allergic response to it and, in some cases, making someone non-allergic to that allergen.

8. Prevention of Allergic Reactions

To prevent or reduce allergic reactions, basic prevention such as dust mite-proof pillowcases and mattresses can help reduce allergens in the bedroom. Additionally, because dust mites multiply quickly in bedding, washing your sheets once a week can be effective. Do make sure to use hot water (130 degrees or higher). Children with severe food allergies should carry injectable epinephrine for emergencies, and anyone with a documented history of anaphylaxis or severe allergic reactions should have two epinephrine auto-injectors available at all times. There are several methods for reducing asthma attacks, based on your specific type of asthma. Generally, pollutants, tobacco smoke, allergens, and viral infections should be prevented. Asthmatics can also use their prescribed long-term controller medication and get an annual influenza vaccine. Florida Allergy & Airways physicians are experienced in treating patients with asthma.

The most effective way to avoid an allergic reaction is to avoid the allergen. This can be done by: 1) avoiding foods you're allergic to if you have food allergies, 2) removing your pet from your home if you're allergic to pet dander, and 3) reducing exposure to pollen by staying indoors during high pollen times (10 a.m. to 4 p.m.) when pollen counts are generally highest. Allergy cleaning products can also minimize your exposure to allergens and prevent or reduce an allergic reaction.

8.1. 1. Avoiding Allergens

Chemicals: Read labels on cleaning products, clothes, or other items. Wearing gloves when handling these items can be a good idea. For more information and suggestions provided by a board-certified allergist, a person may schedule an appointment.

Cockroaches: Since their feces and saliva are what trigger allergies, a safe kitchen can be a good start. As such, it is important to keep all food stored in airtight containers. Crumbs should be cleaned up right away, and garbage should be kept in a can with a tight-fitting lid. Dresses, books, and toys should not be left lying about.

Dust Mites: Covering pillows with casings and mattresses with dust-proof covers can be helpful. Washing bedding regularly in hot water and keeping mattresses and pillows free of allergens can also be beneficial.

Mold: Damp indoor spaces can be a breeding ground for mold. Mold is difficult to completely eradicate from indoor spaces. However, improving ventilation and always running the extractor fan in the bathroom can be helpful. Keep window air conditioners free of moisture and window screens clean.

Avoiding Animals: Dander can be a particular allergen. Regular pet baths, air filters, and cleaning fan blades, walls, and floors can be helpful.

Avoiding Pollen: Check the local news for an idea of the pollen count for any given day. In general, pollen counts are highest between 5 a.m. and 10 a.m. Staying inside when pollen counts are highest and sleeping with the windows closed can be helpful.

If it is known what causes a person's allergic reaction, a doctor may recommend that a person avoids those allergens. In some cases, allergen avoidance can be difficult or impossible. To the extent that it is possible to do so, allergens can be avoided:

8.2. 2. Keeping Living Spaces Clean

Most allergens can be reduced in the home from furniture to clothing. Consider wood floors over carpet, cloth furniture over leather or vinyl, plastic blinds over fabric curtains or drapes, and plastic mattress and pillow covers over cloth. Although beautifying home interiors with curtains or carpets can be done, the more fabric there is the harder it is to eliminate dust from that part of the house and it tends to attract and hold onto allergens easier. Treat your pets like royalty; there's a reason royals wore cloth over leather. Leather and vinyl items for the home are typically easier to clean. While some allergens need to be seen to be treated, regular cleaning ensures there is the least amount of unseen allergens as well. Dusting, vacuuming and washing home goods will remove dust, the allergens that come with it, and maybe some stress while deep cleaning.

While many allergens that cause allergies outdoors may be impossible to eliminate entirely - "you can't get rid of pollen in the air," says - allergens in your home can be reduced by maintaining a clean living space. In fact, this is extremely important for those with allergies because allergens would only otherwise stay in their environment. Keep reading Severe Allergies at School for more information on keeping all kinds of living spaces - including schools - clean, allergy-free environments.

9. Living with Allergies

- Wear protective clothing outdoors. - Avoid wearing sweet-smelling perfumes or scented lotions. - Wear closed-toe shoes when walking outside, especially when you're in wooded or grassy areas. - Consider a medical ID bracelet. If you're allergic to insect stings, it might be a good idea to wear a medical ID bracelet that includes information about your allergy, your doctor, and emergency contacts. - Ask your doctor about allergy shots. People with certain, severe types of allergies can benefit from allergy immunotherapy. This process involves getting a series of allergy shots that help reduce the severity of your hypersensitive reaction to an allergen.

If you have insect sting allergies:

- Eat foods you know are safe. - Check all labels for allergens, even if you don't expect them to appear in a product. - Advocate for yourself. Tell friends and family about your allergies and encourage caretakers to learn everything they can about food allergies. - Join a support group. If you have a food allergy, find a community of people who understand what you're going through. - Understand the FALCPA food-labeling law. Enacted in 2004, this law requires food manufacturers to prominently display any of the "big 8" allergens on a food label. This includes milk, eggs, fish, shellfish, soy, peanuts, tree nuts, and wheat. If a food product contains less than 2% of an allergen, manufacturers don't need to include it in the label.

If you have food allergies:

If your allergies are making daily life a challenge, there are some steps you can take to make things better.

9.1. 1. Allergy Management Tips

Immunotherapy, which is administered via allergy shots or tablets, can reduce the severity of allergic reactions and symptoms. If you have a mild reaction, an antihistamine injection or tablet can help control your symptoms. Eye drops can help with itchy, red, or watery eyes. If you're diagnosed with a mild allergy, you might find it beneficial to consult with a dietitian or nutritionist to learn more about healthy food choices and supplements.

Over-the-counter (OTC) medications are available for a wide range of allergic symptoms, including upset stomachs, sore throats, itchy red eyes, runny noses, skin rashes, and hives. The medications include loratadine, cetirizine, fexofenadine, diphenhydramine, clemastine, ibuprofen, and loratadine. Then, you may require a prescription for corticosteroid nasal sprays, among other medications and treatments, for allergy relief. You may require immunotherapy if your allergies are particularly severe. Ask your doctor for more information.

Medicines

Here are some general allergy management tips: - Try to avoid allergens if possible. Use nasal filters if pollen or irritants are a problem. - Allergy-proof your home. Dust, mold, and pet dander are standard allergens. You can take steps to allergy-proof your house and minimize the impact of these allergens. - Avoid allergy triggers at night by using dust-mite-proof bedding and air conditioning; use high-efficiency air filters. - Keep your house dry. Mold likes damp; therefore, you should minimize the amount of mildew by drying wet areas in your house (ceiling, walls, and floors) and cleaning bathrooms, basements, and kitchens regularly. A range of dehumidifiers can help reduce mold, spores, and dust mites.

Identification and control

Regardless of the type of allergy you suffer from, the symptoms can be unpleasant and affect your life. Understanding your allergy is important for managing it effectively, but you can also take some general steps to minimize the impact of your allergies on your daily life.

Allergy Management Tips

9.2. 2. Support Groups and Resources

There are many allergy non-profit organizations offering free resources. These organizations range in size from the local chapter of The Food Allergy & Anaphylaxis Connection Team (FAACT), which provides advocacy and resources to allergy families, to FARE (Food Allergy Research & Education), a larger organization that hosts conferences and events across the country. The Asthma and Allergy Foundation of America and Allergy and Asthma Network Americas are also large, national resources. These sites offer a cornucopia of background information, including guides to managing allergies within schools and restaurants. FARE, in particular, offers college scholarships for students with allergies and markets to large corporations alongside offering materials for those living with allergies. FARE connects with corporations offering hands-on allergy management and cooking classes that could be helpful.

Isolating experiences can amplify concerns and create stress and anxiety, even for those without allergies. Finding a local or national support group can be beneficial. While meeting others living with the same condition might seem daunting, they will understand exactly what you are going through and may offer helpful tips for allergy management. Additionally, individuals in your local support group may be able to recommend allergy-conscious stores and vendors in your area or other individuals who are educated about and cater to the allergy community. An experienced support group can offer resources, including doctors and allergen-free products. A little time upfront might save you a lot of time and headache in the long run.

Support groups and resources

10. Conclusion and Future Directions

Development of strategies to stimulate and/or elicit regulatory immune response will be increasingly applied by allergists, especially for polysensitized patients. Epigenetics studies will continue to propose factors important for observation of severity of allergic disease. Treatment and prevention New recent medical strategies for the treatment of allergies comprise also and sublingual immunotherapy with aeroallergens and various biological drugs that were just approved for therapy. They specifically target mediators for the diseases and are directed to all next steps in the development of the allergic disease. Further studies will demonstrate the effectiveness and the long-term side effects of those treatments. Also, many studies are validating different prevention strategies for the development of allergies especially in children, which probably influence the development of the disease quite early on in the first few years of life. With each new allergens sensitization problem studies will also have to multiply and wide use some of today's key treatment paths. Interventions preventing the development of new food allergies are underway and currently being evaluated for their cost and decreased disease rate. New technology and understanding of the allergic pathways are soon opening up to new treatment and prevention opportunities.

In conclusion, allergies are becoming increasingly prevalent, particularly in developed and industrialized countries. There are several reasons that this increase may be occurring, including better diagnostic capabilities, keeping environments too clean or reducing beneficial microorganisms (e.g., decreasing exposure to other children, antibiotics), or increasing exposure to airborne pollutants such as pollen or animal dander. Additionally, food allergies and allergic asthma tend to exhibit more severe symptoms and present a larger problem compared to other types of allergic diseases. New diagnostics and therapies require more knowledge of the underlying pathways, which calls for more research focusing on the various forms of allergens and the protective mechanisms.

Common Unhealthy Reactions of the Immune System to Substances

1. Introduction to Unhealthy Reactions of the Immune System

Other parts of the immune system also play a role and make chemicals like histamine to help get rid of allergens that are bothering the person. Some allergens, like pollen or dust, are in the air. Allergens that you swallow are found in foods or medicines. Some allergens you can touch or that can enter your body through your skin. Anaphylaxis is an often severe and sometimes fatal allergic reaction to an allergen. Many Americans are allergic to plants, food, and/or drugs. Unhealthy immune reactions can even hurt some vital body organ systems. These include lungs, nasal passages, throat, and the skin and can lead to such symptoms as coughing, sneezing, congestion, difficulty breathing, itchy eyes, and itchy skin. An allergic reaction to food usually happens quickly or immediately. An overwhelming majority of people with food allergies react to one or more of the top 8 food allergens: cow's milk, tree nuts, peanuts, nuts, soy, fish, crustacean shellfish, and wheat.

Introduction An allergy is when your immune system reacts to a foreign substance, called an allergen. It's an overreaction to something that doesn't bother most others. The result is your body releasing substances to "protect" you. When this happens, the allergic person may have a variety of symptoms. A substance that causes a reaction in an allergic person is called an allergen. The body reacts to an allergen in various ways. One part of the immune system reacts by developing immunoglobulin E (IgE) antibodies. These can cause food allergies and hay fever. The other type of allergy is called cell mediated allergies. These reactions can cause allergic contact dermatitis, allergic reaction to poison ivy, and cause drug reactions. When a person has a food allergy, a very small amount of the food can cause a severe allergic reaction. Magnified images of these cell types are shown in the image below.

1.1. Overview of the Immune System

The tasks of the immune system are to protect against infectious microorganisms, such as viruses and bacteria, to recognize and delete damaged, aged, or dead cells, and to recognize cells that behave in a way that can lead to the development of cancer. The immune system destroys both the cells infected with the organisms (e.g., cells infected with viruses and bacteria) and the infectious microorganisms themselves. The normal immune system is tolerant to nonself and does not destroy healthy tissue. The normal response of the immune system to nonself is to inactivate or "switch off" the immune response when the nonself has been removed. Our natural response to the self is to produce some immune and/or inflammatory response to this tissue because the tissue has aged or been damaged by radiation, hypoxia, toxins, or other agents.

The immune system is a hierarchical system and is divided into two main parts—the innate, or inborn, system and the acquired, or adaptive, system. The innate system is composed of cells such as macrophages, neutrophils, and natural killer cells. It also includes some of the molecules released from cells of the innate system in response to an infection. The acquired system is composed primarily of T and B lymphocytes and their products. These products include antibodies and cytokines released by T cells. Both systems have the ability to distinguish between self and what is foreign—nonself.

1.2. Types of Unhealthy Immune Reactions

Hypersensitivity Reactions - In Big Picture Terms: This text will go through all of these generally, one-by-one, detailing more specifics about them. It is important to keep in mind, though, that many of these occur in concert with each other in any given patient. For example, a Type 3 Hypersensitivity reaction might well be happening at the same time as a Type 5 reaction. Consequently, the overall presentation can be complicated, and it can be misleading to say that a particular damage picture should be caused by one immune reaction rather than another: they frequently coexist to produce what is seen in individual patients.

There are many different ways in which the immune system can react to substances in unhealthy ways. Generally speaking, there are several types of immune reactions that occur in unhealthy (non-protective) ways: (1) Antibody-mediated processes, occurring in fairly short timeframes, based on cells that occur naturally, but exaggerated or altered in specifics; (2) Antigen-antibody complex diseases - not involving directly attacking cells, but leading to a deposit of antigen-antibody complexes, principally in blood vessels; (3) Genetic susceptibility to infection; (4) Immune complex complement activity; (5) Helper T-cell driven processes (Type 4 Hypersensitivity); (6) T-cell mediated allergies (Type 5 Hypersensitivity). As will be seen below, not all of these fit well within these arbitrary categories, but this classification can help as a framework to understand where in the overall scheme the reaction is.

2. Most Common Substances Causing Immune Reactions

The first immunological model is a lupus-like reaction to silica particles; the second model is regional alveolitis in guinea pigs caused by kaolin (deposited under the skin) coated, but not contaminated, with bovine serum albumin. When, at last, the first immunological reactions to airborne allergens were reported, two of the observed fewmologist allergens, i.e. plicatic acid and cypress camphor, acted by chemical irritation of the nose, conjunctiva, or methacholine-suppressive sensitivity, as well as by delayed skin reactions similar to that shown by dacthal (DCPA), several exposure parts of which we banned.

Food is usually suggested as the most likely substance to provoke an adverse immune response, although this was later extended to include other allergens occurring in the air for those whose job it is to deal with them, which led to the diagnosis of allergic alveolitis. For example, two of the most important substances capable of being released in the air around us that are responsible for 90% of the occupational allergens are alpha-amylase and tendamistat; another one is Bacillus subtilis, rarely found in the U.S., but responsible for the cause of our first cluster of the uncommon illness allergic alveolitis at a Bristol workplace. Adverse drug experimental exposures might cause severe lung injury in people, while the use of contact allergens led to observations on benign mechanisms causing easily avoidable lung injury that were investigated by some recent Berkeley workers and can now be prevented.

2.1. Food Allergens

Symptoms of food allergy can occur instantly (after 2 hours or longer) or delayed (1-24 hours after consumption of allergenic foods) and can vary from minor to severe reactions. Recently, food allergy symptoms are not limited to one or more organs, such as the microbiome, metabolism, and skin, but the role of the gastrointestinal system in affecting immune tolerance during the development of food allergies has also been seen. Symptoms of physical reactions to food exposure range from mild to severe, often called one or more of the following: swelling of the tongue, throat and face, rash or hives, pain in the stomach (cramps or diarrhea), vomiting, and asthma are the most severe reactions. Food allergies occur when the immune system overreacts to the consumption of allergens. Immunological responses to allergenic foods can be shown by increased production of allergenic immunoglobulin E (IgE), which will interfere with the activation of defense cells, such as mast cells and basophils. It induces the release of certain proteins from bodies that raise inflammation.

Statistics showed that each year, at least 20% of the world's population will experience allergic disorders, such as DNA allergies, phenotypic family history, and dermal sensitization, of a genetic grant, and the figure is expected to rise by 2% every century. The top 8 food allergens reported to have shown life-threatening reactions worldwide are cow's milk, eggs, cows, wheat, watermelon nuts, soybean grains, and fish. Allergic reactions caused by these top 8 foods (mainly referred to as FA proteins or as FA antigens) are very common in children and adults, and so far, the allergic diagnostic approaches are limited to skin-prick tests, serum-specific chronicity antibodies-CAP, and obtaining a positive oral food challenge (OFC) regarding the allergenic protein.

2.2. Airborne Allergens

There are usually three parts of our body where airborne allergens can cause problems. Talked about in the first section were some of the signs and symptoms of allergic rhinitis. One important point is when all the three parts of the body are affected at the same time PT or ERT in people with asthma may not work right. These categories were general and not all-inclusive to reactions to allergic rhinitis. An airborne allergen is a type of antigen within the body. In many areas, different airborne allergens affect humans. The immune systems of those who spot an airborne allergen as a risk have an unhealthy reaction. The antibodies cause a series of changes that lead to the symptoms of an allergic reaction when an allergen enters the body through the respiratory system. This reaction is called hypersensitivity, which includes the following immune responses: Respiratory tract symptoms.

A lot of substances in the air - or airborne allergens - have the potential to cause immune responses in our bodies. Allergens are found in low levels just about everywhere. Some are considered seasonal allergens, which come from plants flowering at just that particular time of year. Seasonal allergens precede the top of the allergic period, the top would be the highest concentration of allergens "when symptoms are highest," however, some allergens are continuous. Continuous allergens include mite, fungus, animal danders, and certain feathers. The immune reactions that people have to these airborne allergens can be many things including allergic rhinitis and allergic asthma.

2.3. Medications

Therapeutic drugs: antibiotics (antibacterial agents); allopurinol; xanthine oxidase inhibitor, treatment of gout; aminoglycosides antibiotics - amikacin, gentamicin, kanamycin, neomycin, streptomycin, tobramycin. Diagnosis and treatment of life-threatening conditions in hospital and related environments; primarily bactericidal (kills bacteria). Some gram+ as well as most gram- bacteria; include broad-spectrum antibiotics often used in empiric therapy when the precise nature of the infection is unknown. Bactrim = cotrimoxazole - combination drug: trimethoprim/sulfamethoxazole (TMP/SMX) (TMP/SMZ), cotrimoxazole (CTX, Septrin) is a potent drug therapy used in the treatment of many bacterial infections. Bactrim is primarily used in people with AIDS who become ill with a major germ that is typically not dangerous for people who have working immune systems. Pathogen(s): Pneumocystis jiroveci (formerly Pneumocystis carinii) - this Pneumocystis or PJP infection can cause a very severe pneumonia (PCP) in people with weakened immune systems, such as people who have AIDS. Currently, all people with AIDS whose T-cell counts drop below 200 T-cells as a result of HIV coinfection with PJP receive prophylaxis against PJP with SXT. Other medications that may elicit an immune reaction; carbamazepine; Tegretol/Synergy, a seizure medication; hypersensitization; Steven-Johnsons effect; tests for HLA-DQ1 have been identified to the BAI to associated with idiopathic anaphylaxis. These tests are available from LAB CORP (USA) and privately.

With medication, some of the substances that commonly may cause these reactions include antibiotics to biologic drugs. This is not a comprehensive list of medications, drug classes, or chemicals that may cause adverse immune system reactions. At last count, over 300 different drugs and materials used in medical implants or products have been described as associated with so-called "immune-mediated" adverse reactions.

3. Symptoms and Diagnosis of Immune Reactions

3.1. Common Symptoms

3.2. Diagnostic Tests

4. Treatment and Management Strategies

Medications that block the action of the body's histamine response may be beneficial. Antihistamines are effective at managing a plethora of irritable bowel disease symptoms such as weakness, hives, itching, or allergic rhinitis. Flushing and rash may be addressed effectively by mast cell stabilizer and tackifier transportation. It is essential to consult with your doctor if you are considering medication for immune reactions. While over-the-counter antioxidants may alleviate typical muscle three the tingling and/or the facial pressure, other symptoms require medical investigation and diagnosis that may not be responsive to these kinds of initial self-treatment. Oral steroids may be needed in the curtailing to manage anaphylactoid reactions up to the acute allergic reaction.

For those suffering from adverse immune reactions, treatment and management usually involve strategies to control the immune response, avoid triggers, and reduce the likelihood of such a response. Medications, dietary alterations, and avoidance, or specifically designed immunizations may be recommended by your doctor to help manage adverse immune reactions. Desensitization programs through allergen-specific immunotherapy (AIT) may have repetition for allergic responses when practical and safe. Avoidance of substance contact often reduces the initiation of an adverse immune response. Depending upon the extent of reaction to the substance, individuals can find lifestyle and dietary changes significantly reduce the cost of managing allergies long-term. While dietary changes alone may be sufficient for some who have irritable bowel symptoms, medications that manage symptoms are often required for others.

4.1. Medication Options

There are two forms of immunosuppressive drugs: anticoagulants and immunomodulators. Anticoagulants prevent histamine discharge and alleviate symptoms. These often prevent Goblet Cells from forming allergen antibodies. The development of leukotrienes promotes inflammation, constriction of smooth muscles, and the growth of excess mucus. Significant anticoagulants include Guaifenesin, designed to eliminate secretions and allergens, such as Robitussin, Musinex, and Hyomax, the new ones. Immunomodulators may help manage IgE antihistamines, histamines, pulmonary leukotrienes, extra middle state inflammatory mediators, and selective proteins (reduces immunoreactivity). They must be used every day to exercise similar to antihistamines, although not as rapid an effect is achieved for them.

Corticosteroids both short-term and long-term, such as prednisone, can suppress the immune system and minimize allergy symptoms. The treatment can begin with an oral dosage of 1 milligram (mg) per 1 kilogram (kg) of body weight. This dose can subsequently be reduced by half the next day and reduced in half every other day of treatment. Medications such as Zytiga and Xtandi are designed to help prostate cancer patients adjust to both prolonged short-term and chronic reactions. The average treatment duration is 1 to 2 weeks. Certain predispositions, such as high blood pressure, may well exist in you, and the use of corticosteroids needs to be avoided.

4.2. Avoidance Strategies

• Anaphylaxis: Since roughly 50% of fatalities due to anaphylaxis are due to the actions of these medications (e.g., epinephrine, glucagon, steroids), it is important to avoid anaphylactic agents and, thus, further exposure to the antigens. Strict avoidance of the eliciting triggers usually eliminates immediate type food allergic reactions. Keeping the EAI (epinephrine autoinjector) injector treatments within their use-by dates, e.g. by recycling an expired EpiPen with the EpiPens expired two months earlier, and checking occasionally the use-by dates is important. Additionally, keeping an EpiPen or other auto-injector pen near, or in, a separate piece of clothing or backpack or automobile is also a good avoidance strategy, in case the shirt (or the carrying facility) is vomited on or accidentally opens.

• Idiopathic Urticaria: Urticarial individuals cannot avoid the rapid absorption of a substance and the onset of the wheals. However, avoiding potential triggers, or at least reducing contact with triggers to the greatest extent possible, through close observation and trial-and-error is key. Reducing physical skin irritation and heat and seeking shade on sunny days, while working, exercising, or relaxing, is a part of this avoidance strategy. Eating plain pure foods is recommended. In addition, consultation with a doctor to classify and treat the urticaria subtypes is important.

The best strategies for the management of immune reactions are avoidance and reduction. Avoidance strategies depend upon what elicited the food reactions. The following are some steps that individuals with adverse immune reactions to substances can take to either minimize their exposure to the stimuli of the adverse reactions or to minimize any adverse effects from exposure.

4.3. Immunotherapy

At the moment, immunotherapy is still the most common and most effective way of treating immune reactions. A new treatment approach is to use dietary strategies to develop acceptance in the body's immune system in the same way as the breakdown of acceptance is used as a complementary therapy to the conventional treatment. Maybe in the future it will also be possible to specifically inhibit the infestation of autoimmune diseases. Only then would the immune system diseases be healed and not just contain their effects.

Possible Future Strategy for autoimmune diseases

This treatment has the same aim as conventional allergy treatment with corticosteroids or antihistamines. It is based on the principle that there is an alternative state close to tolerance. Very small doses of the triggers are supposed to build up acceptance in the body's immune system. In the very first stages, it may even be necessary to extract immune system cells and modify them before re-injection. This is a time-consuming process, so this therapy form is only being tested at the moment and cannot be used as a routine therapy.

5. Prevention of Immune Reactions

The second strategy aims at the prevention of the first
substantial breakthrough of the disease and the
interruption of its symptomatic onset, which can occur
very early in the lifetime of an individual. Maintenance
doses of specific immunotherapy can be effective in disease
prevention. Since it is known that both the risks and the
benefits of such preventive measures are dose-dependent,
the introduction of specific immunotherapy in the
preventive settings falls within the general debate upon
"preventive doses" in allergen exposure versus
"maintenance doses" in allergen treatment.

In terms of prevention, two potential immunological
approaches against allergic diseases, the onset of an
adverse immune response, have been especially
investigated in the past. The first one addresses the period
directly after contact of an individual with a potentially
allergic substance in order to lower the probability of an
unfavorable immune reaction. Several epidemiologic
studies have provided increasing evidence that early
allergen exposure is a relevant determinant of later allergic
disease, and the translation of such knowledge into
primary preventive measures has been an issue of
enormous interest. The early introduction of allergenic
foods is the most studied of these and, within the last few
years, a couple of interventional studies clearly reached the
bottom line of disease prevention as some of the more
striking highlights. However, further follow-up data are

needed to confirm these early results. One of the most promising approaches, yet a matter of continuing discussion, is the application of controlled prenatal or very early infantile environmental control measures in families at high risk for allergic disease. Notably, long-term interventional studies are needed to obtain insights into the natural history of controlled allergen exposure and to investigate whether these interventions could be protective against asthma and atopic disease.

5.1. Early Introduction of Allergenic Foods

Some foods may trigger immune responses if introduced early in life, but the findings of studies that have tried this approach are not consistent. One possible advantage relates to foods that generally trigger immune responses. The practice of introducing allergenic foods into the diet of babies without sensitivities to that food is based partly on evidence that people who consume their own eggs have lower rates of egg sensitivity and severe allergic reactions. Several studies on infants who ingested milk proteins on skin or within the digestive system found a decreased likelihood of having sensitivity to milk. In some populations, "the earlier the introduction, the better the tolerance measured." This theory was supported by research in which Australian breastfed infants with no allergies were introduced to allergen foods. The researchers discovered a 67 percent drop in allergies as a result of their allergenic characteristics, including peanut, milk, and eggs. Asthma and environmental allergic sensitization risk was decreased by 13% and 7%, respectively.

Research has been conducted to determine the role of early introduction of allergenic foods in preventing the development of immune responses to those substances. As a result, some of the research has found that early introduction of allergenic foods can be beneficial. A similar reduction in risk has been observed when potential allergens such as asthma or environmental (non-food) allergens have been introduced early, although less evidence has been found for other non-food allergens. One strategy to prevent future immune reactions is to promote tolerance and prevent the development of allergies early in life. The exact mechanism of this advantage is not completely understood. This concept is based on the above findings, which have been proven to be beneficial in preventing allergies and immune reactions in young children.

5.2. Environmental Control Measures

Minimizing exposure to agents known to incite or exacerbate asthma and allergic responses or other immune responses in certain individuals is critical to the prevention/amelioration of hypersensitivity-related disorders. Discussions about allergen and adjuvant-reducing strategies could provide practitioners with information about potential verification techniques, use and impact of allergen-reducing devices, and approaches to remove inside environmental allergens from involves dust mites and their feces, animal dander, molds, pollen, insects, feathers, and hairs/epithelial, as well as outdoor allergens that enter the inside through various routes. Application of Toxocara control measures can also lead to the prevention and management of allergic reactivity, given that exposed individuals develop inappropriately strong immune responses. Comfort measures/ingestion avoidance strategies are also discussed, especially for allergenic foods, and will be relevant in controlling aqueous or structured food allergies as well.

Environmental control measures include the development of relatively allergen-free environments, which can be broadly or narrowly targeted, in response to allergic responses. For those with recognized allergies, essentially this means the elimination of personal triggers through sophisticated environmental and occupational history and the utilization of antigen avoidance in healthcare settings. Currently, a commonsense approach to reducing environmental triggers irrespective of the patient's off-the-shelf allergen-sensitization is prudent, based on gold-standard recommendations for avoidance and environmental control.

6. Impact of Immune Reactions on Quality of Life

The emotional state of mind of those affected also plays a central role. Feelings such as despair, helplessness, and anxiety come up, especially during life crises and in some of the severe forms of disease. Depression and a poorer quality of life have also been reported. The income and careers of the vast majority of those affected are at risk. They are more likely to be absent from work and their absence tends to be more prolonged. Their choice of work may also converge, although this is partly due to the chronic nature of many immune reactions involving the substances. Social life and leisure activities are further restricted by participating in various strategies for the prevention and alleviation of symptoms. Many of those affected have trouble getting a good night's sleep. It is often the symptoms of the immune reactions that keep them awake, or they wake several times during the night. Travel and leisure activities are also very restricted.

Reactions by the immune system can take their toll on the quality of life of people who are affected. The nature and degree of these impairments vary considerably depending on the affected person, the substance causing the immune reaction, the organ systems affected, the severity and duration of the disease, and any other existing conditions. Many affected people experience an impairment of their general state of health and vitality. As a result, they often describe their health as poor compared to the rest of the population. According to those affected and their relatives, the physical, emotional, and social consequences of the disease affect everyday life and overall well-being.

7. Research and Future Directions

Overall, the immune system is quite incredible. It evolves over time and reacts to billions of different substances in the environment using the same basic process: acting from detection, to responding, to resolving. However, just like everything else in biology, the immune system isn't perfect. It can sometimes overreact to things people here in the Information Company might think of as more benign, leading to disease. Researchers are constantly exploring the immune system's responses and learning more about how it works. The more that is understood about the sensitivities of the immune system, the prospects exist for making better predictions about who might develop an allergy or sensitivity to a medication. Furthermore, this may lead to the development of new, more effective therapies for individuals experiencing side effects of a medication due to an immune reaction.

Up to this point, I have talked primarily about T cell responses and how those responses lead to disease. I have also just mentioned at a high level that over time, we have developed a better understanding of some of the immune system's responses to small molecules that lead to a health outcome. Research in this space is ongoing, with many exciting advancements. In recent years, the number of total publications describing this area of research has been steadily increasing. Future areas of investigation include the identification of people who react to new medications before they take them, to predict who will get a specific side effect to a medication or who should avoid certain medical therapies based on their immune reaction to the medication. Additionally, efforts are focused on how to reverse these immune responses in a patient population who has already experienced side effects from medications. Currently, there are no therapeutic strategies to reverse or prevent the adverse benchside of medications due to immune response, but a lot of research efforts are focused on advancing knowledge in this space and understanding the limitations of the immune system.